Florian Georg Pichler

Health promotion from an osteopathic perspective

Florian Georg Pichler

Health promotion from an osteopathic perspective

Osteopathy in health promotion using the example of influencing lung function

ScienciaScripts

Imprint

Cover image: www.ingimage.com

This book is a translation from the original published under ISBN 978-3-330-51415-7.

Publisher:
Sciencia Scripts
is a trademark of
Dodo Books Indian Ocean Ltd. and OmniScriptum S.R.L publishing group

120 High Road, East Finchley, London, N2 9ED, United Kingdom
Str. Armeneasca 28/1, office 1, Chisinau MD-2012, Republic of Moldova, Europe
Managing Directors: Ieva Konstantinova, Victoria Ursu
info@omniscriptum.com

Printed at: see last page
ISBN: 978-620-2-37546-7

Table of contents

CHAPTER 1

Introduction

"To find health should be the object of the practitioner; anyone can find disease." A. T Still, founder of osteopathy (Stone, 2002).

Osteopathy is understood as a science, art and philosophy (Gibbons, 2004) that is applied to people of all ages for health promotion, prevention and rehabilitation.

Osteopathy is an alternative healing method and is now taught as a patient-centred approach (WHO, 2014).

Osteopathy can achieve its greatest effect in strengthening health, particularly in prevention, which aims to eliminate risk factors (Steinbach, 2007).

I have been interested in health promotion and prevention for several years and have already been involved in projects in cooperation with Univ. Prof. Dr Hans Tilscher (www.ortho-motion.com) to help shape workplace health promotion.

In these projects, particular attention was paid to the "low tech high touch instead of high tech low touch" approach. Osteopathic manual functional examination techniques and the assessment of structural and functional disorders were implemented with a high degree of importance in these projects.

The identification of respiratory dysfunction was also given high priority in the assessment of health status.

In order to reinforce the role of osteopathy in the healthcare system and in prevention, there is a need to strengthen the evidence base on the effectiveness of osteopathy.

Recent calculations show that the use of osteopathy results in lower costs for health insurance companies and thus significant potential savings (Ismail-Tsaous, 2014).

Through comprehensive anamnesis and detailed physical examination, osteopathy offers the possibility of individualised and cost-effective treatment. Bio-psycho-social factors are taken into account, thus holistically assessing the resources available to the individual.

The increasing number of lung diseases such as COPD and allergies (Associations, 2015) also makes it particularly important to look into effective therapeutic approaches that can improve the functionality of the respiratory system.

Several master's theses have already addressed the topic of the effect of osteopathy on lung function, e.g. in firefighters and athletes. Positive trends regarding the immediate effect of osteopathy on lung function have been identified (Hellich, The immediate influence of osteopathy on the respiratory performance of firefighters, 2011) (Böhmüller, 2007).

Chaitow (Chaitow L., 2004) also sees relevance in detecting and eliminating respiratory dysfunctions for the effective treatment of low back pain (LBP).

Further studies have investigated the effect of osteopathy on lung function and lung disease (Donald R. Noll,

Brian F. Degenhardt, Jane C. Johnson, & Selina A. Burt, 2008). The authors unanimously agreed that the duration and number of techniques used should be limited and that an individual approach to treatment is recommended (Donald R. Noll, Brian F. Degenhardt, Christian Fossum, & Kendi Hensel, 2008).

An improvement in lung function in a healthy population has already been demonstrated with a single technique. In this randomised placebo-controlled study with a total of 40 people per group, a significant (p< 0.05) improvement between the pre- and post-test FEV1 (forced expiratory volume in 1 second) values in a spirometer follow-up examination after 5 and 20 minutes (Francisco Jose Gonzales-Alvarez, 2014).

This study by Gonzales-Alvarez motivated me to try to reproduce this significant effect through the application of time-limited but individually tailored osteopathic treatment.

The aim of this study was therefore to investigate the effect of osteopathy on the respiratory system of healthy individuals, with a particular focus on lung function and subjective perception of exertion.

CHAPTER 2

Prevention and health promotion

The terms prevention and health promotion are often not clearly distinguished from one another or are used synonymously. The following paragraphs attempt to clarify these terms.

The root of the term "prevention" comes from the Latin word "praevenire" (to forestall). Prevention refers to individual and societal strategies and measures aimed at avoiding a deterioration in health (Rosenbrock & Gerlinger, 2006).

It can be added that prevention aims to avoid the occurrence of diseases (Klaus, Theodor, & Jochen, 2014).

The term health promotion is considerably younger (Froom & Benbassat, 2000) and was established as a concept of health promotion in Ottawa in 1986 (WHO, Ottawa Charter, 1986).

Based on this concept from Ottawa, Austria also introduced its own Health Promotion Act in 1998.

The Healthy Austria Fund (FGÖ) has taken on the task of raising the profile of health promotion and increasing awareness of it. Health promotion has thus become a central concern of the national health objectives (Health, 2015).

In contrast to prevention, health promotion is about improving living conditions and strengthening opportunities for health development (Klaus, Theodor, & Jochen, 2014).

In the author's view, this apt description of health promotion is particularly consistent with the osteopathic approach to health and illness (see chapter Health and illness from an osteopathic perspective).

2.1 Economic aspects

The Austrian healthcare system is one of the best in the world, but also one of the most expensive.

In 2011, for example, 32.4 billion or, in other words, almost 4,000 euros per capita was spent (Health, 2015, p. 19).

Older figures indicate that all health insurance providers had already accumulated a deficit of €253 million by 2004 (Hofmarsch & Rack, 2015).

Like many other countries, Austria is facing an ageing population, which is due to both higher life expectancy and a decline in the fertility rate. According to forecasts by Statistics Austria, the Austrian population will grow to over 9 million by 2030.

In 2011, the average number of children was approximately 1.4 per woman, with an average fertility age of 28.5 years. Today, a newborn girl in Austria has a life expectancy of 83.4 years and a newborn boy has a life expectancy of 78.1 years (Health, 2015, pp. 2-3).

In addition to this demographic change, it should also be borne in mind that it will become necessary to remain healthy in the workplace for longer, thereby shifting the age-specific employment rate towards a higher age.

Musculoskeletal disorders are a particularly significant cost factor for the economy, as they are one of the most common causes of pain in industrialised countries. The majority (85%) of these are non-specific spinal complaints. These disorders were already the reason for most sick days in Austria in 2011, with a total of almost 40 million sick days, or in other words, a good 3 million people on sick leave per year (Tilscher, 2015).

On average, people with diseases and disorders of the musculoskeletal system are absent from work for 21.3 days per year (Knieps, 2015).

In searching for the position of osteopathy in the field of health promotion and prevention, the author has come across a number of paradigms in the health system and medicine in general that should be reconsidered and are addressed in the following chapter, Paradigm shifts in health policy and medicine.

2.2 Paradigm shifts in health policy and medicine

It is well known that political strategies are slow to change as a result of new reforms. It should also be noted that osteopathy has been known in Austria since the early 1990s, but is still not legally regulated as a profession or treatment method.

Despite well-founded training programmes for osteopaths in Austria, their integration into the primary health care (PHC) debate is still completely unclear.

In Germany, a recent resolution passed at the German Medical Association conference in Frankfurt in mid-May 2015 clearly shows that, despite the academisation of osteopathy, there is opposition to dividing direct access (e.V., 2015).

In order to give future osteopaths who wish to gain a foothold in public health issues such as health promotion and prevention more skills, consideration should also be given to increasing the number of hours or ECTS (European Credit Transfer System) in the curriculum.

Sweden and New Zealand are exemplary in this respect, having already allocated 15-30 ECTS credits for this in basic physiotherapy training (Swonar, 2015).

Despite its more than 100-year history, osteopathy is in many ways consistent with important strategies for the medicine of the future.

The following table (Table 1) highlights the necessary changes in paradigms of contemporary medicine and future medicine and compares them.

Table 1: Paradigm shift (own representation) from (Bortz, 2011, p. 204)

Current Medicine	**Next Medicine / Medicine of the future**
Disease	Health
Repair / Rehabilitation	Prevention / Health Promotion
External locus of control	Internal locus of control
Structure	Function
Component	System
Episode	Process
High tech	Low tech
Specialist	Primary contact
Rights	Responsibility
Business	Profession / Vocation

Fossum adds that these proposals for the medicine of the future are already very much in line with osteopathic theories, ways of thinking and methods of intervention (Fossum, 2015).

The next table (Table 2) is supplemented with a comparison of conventional medicine and complementary medicine, which also includes osteopathy.

The following table is not exhaustive but serves only as an example to illustrate this line of thought.

Table 2: Criteria for differentiation (own representation) (Liem, 2008, p. 12)

Conventional medicine	**Complementary medicine**
General	individual
objective	Subjective
reproducible	unique
findings	state of mind
Negate and eliminate chance and placebo	Use chance and placebo
Responsibility of the doctor	Responsibility of the patient
Suppression of bodily reactions	Treatment through cooperation with nature
Separation of body, mind and soul	Body, mind and soul form an interacting unit
Matter	Energy
Acute and chronic illnesses are considered separately and independently of each other	Acute illness: attempt to restore homeostasis; chronic illnesses: failed attempts

Liem notes that this polarising table is only partially correct, as osteopathy also sometimes uses conventional medical approaches. For example, therapy does not exclusively stimulate regulatory processes through the use of manual treatment approaches, but also suppresses undesirable symptoms through the use of antagonistic approaches if necessary (Liem, 2008, pp. 11-12).

CHAPTER 3

Osteopathic principles and models

All basic osteopathic principles are closely linked to the concepts of health maintenance and disease management (WHO, The Forum for Osteopathy Regulation in Europe, 2014).
When osteopathy is applied, osteopathic philosophies, principles and structure-function relationship models are also applied (Seffinger, et al., 2011). This has also been comprehensively documented in a standard work on osteopathy:

"Osteopathy (historically osteopathy) is a philosophy, a science and an art. Its philosophy encompasses the concept of the unity of structure and function of the living organism in health and disease. Its science encompasses biological, behavioural, chemical, physical and spiritual knowledge related to the maintenance and restoration of health, as well as the recognition, prevention, cure and alleviation of disease. Its art is the application of philosophy in the practice of medicine and surgery in all its branches and specialities" (Ward, 2003).

For non-medical osteopaths, the Glossary of Osteopathy also provides a definition of osteopathy as a therapy: "Osteopathic manipulative therapy (OMTh)" followed by the following quote:

"The therapeutic application of manually directed forces by an osteopath (non-physician) to improve physiological function and homeostasis impaired by somatic dysfunction" (Osteopathic, 2011).

At this point, the traditional osteopathic principles should be reiterated so that, from the author's point of view, the obvious connections between the concept of health promotion and these principles become clear to the reader (own translation):

- The body is a unit
- Structure influences function
- The law of the artery is essential
- The body has the power to heal and regulate itself (Parson, 2006, pp. 8-9).

These principles can be better understood with the following additions:

- When normal adaptability is disrupted or when environmental factors exceed the body's self-regulatory powers, illness can arise
- The free circulation of bodily fluids is essential for maintaining health
- Nerves play an essential role in controlling fluids in the body
- There are physical conditions that should not only be regarded as part of the disease, but ly also contribute to maintaining the disease state (Parson, 2006, p. 9).

These principles naturally have a strong philosophical character, which is why the five typical structural function models are used in the practical application of osteopathic manual therapy. In practical work, these often serve as working hypotheses.

The following models are intended to help osteopaths correctly classify and evaluate the information they have gathered in order to draw conclusions about the general state of health of their patients (WHO, 2014).

- Biomechanical model
- Neurological model
    a. The autonomic nervous system
    b. The pain concept
    c. The neuroendocrine concept
- Model of respiration and circulation
- Bioenergetic model
- Psychobehavioural model (Gibbons, 2004, pp. 36–37) (Greenman, 1998, pp. 64–67)

As a rule, several of these models can be applied simultaneously to patients, whereby it is necessary for osteopaths to weigh up these models.

Osteopaths should consider both traditional principles and structural-functional models as a framework concept, but above all be aware that all patients with their signs and symptoms represent an interaction of physical, psychological and environmental factors. The importance of the patient-therapist relationship is also an essential part of the therapeutic process. It should therefore be understood as a patient-centred rather than a disease-centred approach (WHO, 2014, p. 3).

In order to correctly contextualise these working hypotheses together with the patient's history, it is necessary to organise all knowledge correctly with the help of clinical reasoning (see Clinical reasoning).

In order to identify the physical components of these models, osteopaths use the concept of somatic dysfunction, which is now explained below.

3.1.1 Somatic dysfunction

The General Osteopathic Council (GOsC) uses the following concise statement as a working hypothesis: Osteopathy is what osteopaths do and somatic dysfunction is what osteopaths find (Parson, 2006).

The Glossary of Osteopathic Terminology describes somatic dysfunction as follows:

"Impaired or altered function of related components of the somatic (physical) system: skeletal, joint and myofascial structures and the associated vascular, lymphatic and neural elements. Somatic dysfunction can be treated with osteopathic manipulation techniques" (AAOM, 2011).

In osteopathy, it is believed that local disturbances or lesions of the musculoskeletal system can severely impair the body's ability to recover (Gibbons, 2004, p. 3).

An essential means of identifying somatic dysfunction is T.A.R.T. (tissue texture change; asymmetry; Restriction of Motion; Tenderness) (Kuchera & Kuchera, 1994, p. 19) or, as Greenman describes, A.B.G (asymmetry; range of motion; tissue texture and Gibbons further expanded with tissue sensitivity (Gibbons,

2004, p. 5).
Somatic dysfunction is particularly evident in the spine. A whole range of signs can be found there: hypertonia of the paravertebral muscles around the affected segment, sympathicotonia of the segment, nerve conduction is affected and lowers the stimulus threshold of all receptors in that area. Thus, persistent somatic dysfunction can be a contributing factor to the chronicity of a problem. Essentially, this highlights the importance of the nervous system as a control and coordination centre and underlines that the spine is very important for diagnosis and therapy (Richter & Hebgen, 2007).
This explanation makes it clear that the concept of somatic dysfunction is similar in many respects to that described in the chapter Normal breathing patterns – dysfunctional breathing patterns.

3.1.2 Health and illness from an osteopathic perspective

Basically, it can be said that against the historical background of the last hundred years, the osteopathic view of health and disease has changed.
This is not least due to the fact that people used to die a hundred times more often from influenza, tuberculosis and pneumonia, for example. Today, people in industrialised countries mainly die as a result of their lifestyle habits, such as stimulants (e.g. tobacco, alcohol), obesity, lack of exercise and stress, to name but the most important (Osborn & Jerome, 2011).

In Austria, the top three causes of death are cardiovascular disease, followed by cancer and respiratory diseases (Gesundheit, 2015, p. 5).

In osteopathy, the definitions of health and illness are closely linked to the state of homeostasis, which is equivalent to a harmonious interaction at all bio-psycho-social levels (Hinkeltheim & Zalpour, 2006).
Stone adds (own translation) to the concept of homeostasis that adaptability is an essential characteristic for maintaining health. By this she means that in order to stay healthy, the body must establish a balance between the emotional, chemical and physical environment, knowing full well that the body itself consists of mental, physical and chemical components. From this, it can be concluded that homeostasis is not a rigid situation but describes a state in which constant exchange is possible in order to ultimately return to a normal level (Stone, 2002, pp. 15-17).
Dr. Still often compared humans to a machine that had been perfectly developed by nature or an intelligent creator ( ). This perfect machine, the human body, does not need any external medicine, but contains all the substances necessary to produce and maintain health (Stark, 2007).
To provide an important anchor for the definition of health, the WHO definition is quoted below:

"Health *is a state of complete physical, mental and social well-being and not merely the absence of disease or infirmity" (WHO, Constitution, 1946).*

A panel of osteopathic experts assembled by Torsten Liem and Peter Sommerfeld does not entirely agree with this distinction between health and illness:
Sommerfeld states that this definition is too idealistic and places excessive demands on therapists. Complete

health is equated with a successful life, and doctors and therapists are then held responsible for this. Health cannot be separated from illness, and even death cannot ultimately be excluded. Kaschowitz expands on this statement by pointing out that illness is a social phenomenon (Nagel, 2008).

In his master's thesis, Risch identified the following as the most important concepts of health for German-speaking osteopaths with an academic background:

Health as a sensory experience followed by
health as a sociological experience,
health as change or transformation,
health as connection, and
health as experience (Risch, 2015, p. 5).

The following quote from Dr Still in Kuchera concludes this section:

"Dr. Still's idea of health was a body in which all parts and structures work together as perfectly as possible, a mind and a soul, all living together in an environment that provides all the necessary conditions for life. This is the principle of unity of the body" (Kuchera & Kuchera, 1994).

CHAPTER 4

The respiratory system

In order not to go beyond the scope of this paper, further explanations of the respiratory system will be limited to the subcomponents of respiratory mechanics and respiratory pattern dysfunction.
The respiratory system refers to the entire system of organs responsible for breathing. The physiological function of the lungs is gas exchange, i.e. the uptake of oxygen into the body and the release of carbon dioxide from the body. (Zalpour, 2006, pp. 429-441).

4.1 Respiratory mechanics

The movement of the lungs is largely determined by the width of the thorax, i.e. the position of the ribs and the dynamics of the diaphragm.
Respiratory mechanics comprise inspiration and expiration and occur approximately 10 to 15 times per minute in adults and up to 25 times per minute in children. This ventilates the alveolar spaces with oxygen-rich air and expels carbon dioxide-rich, oxygen-poor air. Since the lungs are elastic and do not move actively themselves, they follow the movement of the thorax due to the negative pressure in the pleural cavity (Zalpour, 2006, pp. 417–431).

Breathing not only influences homeostatic functions, but also systems such as the autonomic nervous system, the cardiovascular system, and chemical and other metabolic regulations. In addition, breathing has an influence on motor control and posture (Courtney, 2009).
Kuchera explains in more detail:

"Breathing is a dynamic process involving reflexes, nerve activity, the diaphragmatic muscles and various other muscles, as well as the movement of the fasciae and an estimated 146 joints in the body. The efficiency of this interaction is necessary for effective inhalation and exhalation, respiration and the creation of pressure gradients between the chest and abdominal cavities. The cyclical pressure gradients act like a pump for the lymphatic system and promote good lymph and venous flow as well as the physical reactions that take place in the bloodstream during breathing" (Kuchera & Kuchera, 1994).

This complex sub-function of the body can be thrown out of balance by a variety of mechanisms. These include, among other things, sources of disturbance such as biomechanical mobility impairments of the thorax, diaphragm function, neurological causes and viscerofacial disorders. The most important of these, in the author's view, are considered and briefly explained in the following chapters on the myofascial system and the visceral system.

4.1.1 Normal breathing patterns – dysfunctional breathing patterns

Normal diaphragmatic breathing consists of a slower breathing rate (6-8 breaths per minute) with a volume of >2000 ml (Peper & Tibbetts, 2015).
The normal breathing pattern is characterised by air flowing through the nose and throat, passing through the

larynx and into the lungs during inspiration. The diaphragm descends so far that the abdominal wall bulges forward. The upper part of the chest and the auxiliary breathing muscles remain relaxed. Exhalation occurs without any effort by the diaphragm, which returns to its dome-shaped starting position, supported by the elastic recoil of the lungs. This is followed by a relaxed pause during which the diaphragm readjusts itself for the next cycle. In summary, it can be said that normal breathing patterns are barely perceptible and can quickly become economical again even after physical or emotional states (Bradley D., 2002, p. 44).

The term breathing pattern includes the location of dominant breathing movements (chest or abdominal breathing), the presence or absence of upper trunk muscle activity, the timing and flow rate of breathing during inhalation and exhalation, and the pauses between breaths. These breathing patterns can also be found in phrases such as "take a breath", "a sigh of relief", "my breath catches", "be out of breath", "gasp for air" and "be inspired". These expressions reflect the mind-body relationships in which breathing patterns influence the body and vice versa (Peper & Tibbetts, 2015).

Breathing Pattern Disorders (BPD) or Dysfunctional Breathing describe a combination of altered breathing patterns and hyperventilation and are best translated as dysfunctional breathing patterns in German-speaking countries. Dysfunctional breathing patterns can range from a mild form of high-chest breathing to a severe form known as hyperventilation syndrome (Chaitow L., Physiopedia, 2015).
Breathing patterns are often hidden and conditioned by habitual and normal activities. These conditioned patterns include holding your breath when the phone rings, shallow chest breathing when typing on a computer, and heavy breathing during a speech (Peper & Tibbetts, 2015).
It is estimated that dysfunctional breathing patterns affect approximately 10% of the population. It has been noted that women (14%) are significantly more affected than men (2%) (Thomas, McKinley, Freeman, & Foy, 2005).

Breathing pattern dysfunctions are particularly noticeable when breathing is no longer effective enough or when the affected person is no longer able to respond adequately to environmental conditions or physical circumstances (Courtney, 2009).
A number of authors have already addressed the various facets of this dysfunction. The psychological and physical reactions are highlighted by osteopath Chaitow, who also points out the frequency of this functional disorder of the respiratory mechanism in his book "Multidisciplinary Approaches to Breathing Pattern Disorders" (Chaitow Leon, 2002).
The following description provides a good insight into the complexity of this particular dysfunction:

"Dysfunctional breathing (DB) is defined as chronic or recurrent changes in breathing patterns that cannot be attributed to a specific medical diagnosis and lead to respiratory and non-respiratory complaints. It is not a disease process in the sense of a " " but merely changes in breathing patterns that impair normal respiratory processes. Breathing disorders are holistic problems, especially in long-term illnesses, where dysfunctional breathing can destabilise the mind and muscles, mood and metabolism. They can play a role, for example, in premenstrual syndrome, chronic fatigue, neck, back and pelvic pain, fibromyalgia and some aspects of anxiety and depression" (Chaitow Leon, 2002).

All these consequences lead to a massive increase in stress for patients and place an unnecessary burden on the healthcare system. All too often, this syndrome is not yet identified. As a result, patients with alarming symptoms regularly come to the emergency room and, after serious pathologies have been ruled out, are labelled as overly anxious. This means that no further therapy recommendations are made for the treatment of the dysfunctional breathing pattern (Bradley D., 2002, pp. 43-60).

If insufficient exhalation occurs on a permanent basis, a state of hypocapnia ensues (hypocapnia describes a reduced partial pressure of carbon dioxide in the arterial blood) (Wikipedia, Wikipedia The Free Encyclopaedia, 2015). This hypokapnia can occur, for example, with rapid and/or deep breathing, known as hyperventilation, or with respiratory compensation of metabolic acidosis (exhalation of acid valences) (Chin, et al., 2007).

Hyperventilation can be divided into acute and chronic forms. In the acute form, the dysfunctional breathing pattern of hyperventilation manifests itself in deep and rapid breathing and the distinct use of the upper thoracic respiratory muscles. Oxygen saturation is normal and patients appear to be clearly agitated or stressed (Bradley D., 2002, p. 47).

The chronic form of this breathing pattern dysfunction is much more difficult to diagnose. Patients with this form of the disorder usually only come to attention when there is a new acute episode or when all other special examinations have failed to produce any results (Bradley D., 2002, p. 43-60).

In a further study, Bradley and colleagues found that individuals who performed poorly on a standardised movement screening test were more likely to have breathing pattern dysfunction (hyperventilation syndrome) and also exhibited muscular imbalance and disturbances in muscular control (Bradley & Esformes, 2014). This shows that some key structures must function smoothly, which will be discussed in the chapter on the myofascial system and the visceral system.

4.1.2 Myofascial system and visceral system

Structures such as the diaphragm, the fascial system, the visceral system and the nervous system play a major role in relation to dysfunctional breathing patterns.

Many of the characteristics of the diaphragm reflect some of the functions of the respiratory system mentioned above.

Gas exchange in the lungs is regulated by the inspiratory and expiratory movements of the diaphragm. The organs are moved by the rhythmic change in pressure, stimulating diffusion and osmosis processes with , as well as drainage and dilation of the sinus venosus of the skull and the jugular veins. The diaphragm helps maintain stability in the torso, thereby facilitating movement of the extremities. Not to be forgotten are the vascular and neural structures that pass through the diaphragm. Due to its diverse functions, the diaphragm is very often dysfunctional (Richter & Hebgen, 2007, pp. 88-89).

In visceral osteopathy, it is known that fasciae connect different tissues and react as a unit to disruptive factors. Disruptions in fascia dynamics can therefore influence the haemodynamic and neurovegetative function of organs (Hebgen, 2008, p. 16).

In a healthy or normal person, there is a physiological increase in pressure in the abdominal cavity, with a value of around 5-7 mm HG. Finet and William further explain that any dysfunction of the diaphragm and an increase in pressure in the abdominal cavity impede blood flow in the abdominal cavity and the lymphatic system. The consequences can be seen as far as the femoral vein and the portal vein, with reduced flow rates (Finet & William, 2012, p. 16).

Some studies have shown that the visceral abdominal organs, in particular the upper abdominal organs, perform continuous and predictable movements during breathing. In people between the ages of 25 and 65 in an upright position, all organs descend in the sagittal plane during inhalation (Finet & Williame, 2012, p. 16-18).

In addition to post-operative reasons that influence a change in visceral mobility and increased abdominal pressure, incorrect muscle activation sequences can also contribute to this. The following muscle systems that have a postural and respiratory function, such as the diaphragm, transverse abdominis muscle and pelvic floor muscles, can be affected in their ability to activate by low back pain and iliosacral pain syndromes. The ability to activate these muscles may also be affected on one side only (Finet & Williame, 2012, p. 20).

Ever since Litteljohn established the biomechanical model of lines of force (Richter & Hebgen, 2007, pp. 58-59), conclusions about disorders of the viscerofascial system can be drawn from a precise inspection of posture. A distinction can be made between anterior, posterior and centred posture patterns (Corts, 2012).

Typical postural stereotypes include:

- shortened trunk extensors,
- a stiff thoracolumbar transition,
- poor pelvic control,
- restricted hip extension and

excessive axial rotation lead to dysfunctional breathing patterns and pelvic floor insufficiency (Key, 2007). This makes it clearer that it will not always be possible to identify a primary lesion.

Osteopaths must correctly interpret these complex exemplary relationships in order to arrive at an osteopathic diagnosis or hypothesis and develop a treatment plan. This analytical, academic approach will be discussed in more detail in the following chapter, Clinical reasoning .

In this context, it should be noted that in osteopathy, the relevance of intuition (= the ability to gain insight into facts, perspectives, laws or the subjective consistency of decisions without conscious conclusions) (Wikipedia, 2015) should not be neglected. Sidler adds that, despite its high relevance, there is hardly any osteopathic literature on this subject (Sidler, 2010).

4.1.3 Clinical reasoning

Clinical reasoning is now an integral part of osteopathy and osteopathic training. In simple terms, the term could be translated as reflective thinking or clinical reasoning (Batrow, 2012).

Fr Fink-Koller devoted her master's thesis to this topic several years ago, in which she produced an excellent synthesis of traditional philosophical osteopathic approaches and clinical reasoning.

"This way of thinking is used in osteopathy, manual therapy and medicine to form preliminary hypotheses

after taking the patient's medical history and performing a physical examination, and then to make a diagnosis. This allows the practitioner to choose the appropriate form of treatment that confirms or refutes the previously established hypotheses, depending on how the treatment affects the patient. Therapeutic thinking aims to solve specific problems by achieving a transition from the current state (e.g. headache) to a desired state (freedom from symptoms). Thinking about possible activating factors leads to specific actions in the form of therapeutic treatment approaches" (Fink-Koller, 2015).

Oliver Thompson, an English osteopath working in the field of science, and his colleagues have made a significant contribution to the analysis and identification of osteopaths' attitudes and approaches to clinical reasoning strategies.
Two apt quotes emerge from this work:

"The clinical thinking processes that lead to the establishment of a diagnosis are fundamental to safe, effective and efficient clinical practice and are central to professional autonomy and accountability. While research has identified the diagnostic reasoning approaches of a range of health professions, there is limited understanding of how osteopaths make diagnoses in clinical practice" (Thomson, Petty & Moore, 2014).

"Clinical reasoning is an integral part of clinical practice and, for osteopaths, involves more than just formulating a diagnosis. With the advent of evidence-based practice, health professionals are required to disclose the strategies behind their clinical decisions. As many other health professions critically examine their practice models, the profession of osteopathy also has the same need to reflect on and improve the transparency of the clinical practice models used in osteopathy" (Thomson, Petty & Moore, 2011).

In summary, it can be said that consistent reflection and analysis of the patient data and information collected is an important aspect of osteopathy, although it should be emphasised once again that the importance of intuition should not be overlooked.
The next chapter presents the scientific work on the effects of osteopathy on the respiratory system and a selection of appropriate examination steps and measures.

CHAPTER 5

Osteopathy for the respiratory system

The following chapter provides a brief overview of osteopathic techniques and the effects of osteopathy. Finally, the most important assessment methods are described, followed by a description of placebo and sham treatments in the context of osteopathic research.

5.1 Study situation and measures

The professional approach is generally considered to be selecting the appropriate osteopathic measures after examining the patient.

However, an expert interview with ten osteopaths concluded that although a standardised approach to examination was considered important, there was no significant disagreement in the choice of tests and starting position during the examination itself (Biberschick, 2015).

For the present study, an attempt was therefore made to provide a rough checklist for the treating osteopath. Based on the treatment region and treatment approaches described in the study by Noll (2008), these were mapped out (see Appendix A).

Upon critical examination of the published osteopathic literature, the author believes that there are clear trends towards assigning certain osteopathic techniques to individual clinical pictures and/or diseases or patient groups. This seems to be a logical consequence of the proven effectiveness of individual techniques.

As already explained in the previous chapters, the interconnection between breathing and the visceral and fascial systems as well as the neurological system is particularly strong. These facts underline how important it is to ensure smooth breathing movements in almost every disease (Willard, 2011).

Measures that have been found in the literature to have an influence on the respiratory system include the "rib raising technique", which influences lung function by stimulating the sympathetic nervous system in patients with or without asthma (Wheatley, Gosling, & Gibbons, 2000).

It should be noted that the speed at which the technique is performed has a significant influence on its effectiveness. An Australian research group was able to show that a rapidly performed "rib raising technique" triggered the greatest increase in respiratory rate in a group of healthy subjects. They attributed this to a particularly strong activation of the sympathetic nervous system (Farthing, Gosling, Williams, & Vaughan, 2006).

Further techniques were investigated, some as individual techniques.

A pilot study on the effect of osteopathic diaphragmatic release techniques and intercostal stretching on oxygen saturation after physical activity on a cross trainer showed no effect on oxygen saturation compared to no intervention (Goyal, 2015).

Another study investigating the effect of diaphragmatic release and rebound techniques found a positive trend towards improved thoracic mobility in a group of 41 healthy individuals, but this was not statistically significant (Dennison, 2015).

As already described in the introduction, an improvement in lung function in a healthy population has already been demonstrated with a single technique. In this randomised placebo-controlled study with a total of 40 people per group, a significant (p< 0.05) improvement between the pre- and post-test FEV1 (forced expiratory volume in 1 second) values in a spirometer follow-up examination after 5 and 20 minutes (Francisco Jose Gonzales-Alvarez, 2014).

5.2 Assessments

Osteopathic philosophy and models used for the examination have already been discussed. The question of suitable assessment tools to prove the effect and effectiveness of therapy is increasingly being raised in all health professions.
The problem that arises time and again is that the majority of diagnostic procedures (e.g. imaging, MRI, X-ray, blood analysis) are aimed at finding pathological and/or structural changes and that the importance of a good clinical examination is forgotten (Buckup, 2009).
The concepts of somatic dysfunction and dysfunctional breathing patterns refer to functional changes that are often only temporary. Therefore, attempts are usually made to collect subjective and objective parameters in order to at least indirectly prove the existence of a dysfunction.

5.3 Placebo versus osteopathic interventions

In order to prove the effectiveness of osteopathic manual therapy, one must adhere to current standards. This includes choosing an optimal research design in the sense of an RCT (randomised controlled trial). A decision must be made in favour of a placebo or sham treatment. This is necessary in order to identify a difference between the chosen intervention and the control treatment. The big challenge here is to choose a measure that the patients also expect to have a therapeutic effect. Fulda examined the expectations of patients from three interventions: HVLA, light touch and ultrasound applications. She concluded that the expectations for ultrasound were most similar to those for HVLA (Kimberly G Fulda, 2007). Lougee also believes that the use of a non-active physical instrument as a comparison to manual interventions proves to be useful (Hannah Lougee, 2013).
Janine Leach appeals for the development of an osteopathic concept for evaluating evidence in the future. Patients should not be involved in the work as subjects but as active scientists (Leach, 2008).
Within the scope of this study, a physical device, a non-active microwave, was therefore used for the " " (MOPSE) application. For further information, see the chapter on test materials. The single osteopathic treatment and the placebo treatment were defined as lasting 15 minutes. This time unit was already recommended in the MOPSE Multicenter Osteopathy Pneumonia Study in the Elderly protocol (Donald R. Noll, Brian F. Degenhardt, Christian Fossum, & Kendi Hensel, 2008).
The methods used in this study are essentially classic osteopathic measures. Parietal, visceral and craniosacral techniques were used. The treating osteopath selected the methods necessary to resolve the somatic dysfunctions found. These included the following special measures: impulse techniques, soft tissue techniques and fascial techniques, muscle energy techniques and positional release techniques, as well as long lever techniques, techniques on the omentum maj.et min, radix techniques, grand abdominal manoeuvres, doming diaphragm, rib raising and occiput release techniques. For a detailed description of these techniques and measures, please refer to the standard works by Greenman and Ward (Greenman, 1998)

(Ward, 2003).

CHAPTER 6

Research question

Can osteopathic treatment immediately change subjective physical performance and lung function in healthy adults?

The PICOT scheme was used to develop the research question.
Population: The study group consisted of young healthy adult men and women, i.e. students in their second semester of a physiotherapy degree programme.
Intervention: All classic osteopathic manual therapy measures (parietal, visceral and craniosacral) tailored to the individual based on the findings.
Control intervention: A placebo treatment with an inactive microwave was used.
Outcome: What measurable influence does osteopathy have on the respiratory system?
Time: A single intervention involving placebo and osteopathic treatment was evaluated for effectiveness before and after the intervention.

6.1 Null hypothesis HO

There is no difference between an intervention group (osteopathic treatment) and a control group (placebo treatment) after a step test in terms of the lung function value FEV1.

6.2 Alternative hypothesis H1

There is a difference between an intervention group (osteopathic treatment) and a control group (placebo treatment) after a step test in terms of the lung function value FEV1.

6.3 Side hypothesis 02

There is no difference between an intervention group (osteopathic treatment) and a control group (placebo treatment) in terms of the RPE (Rating of Perceived Exertion) of the participants' cardiopulmonary exertion.

6.4 Sub-hypothesis 03

There is no difference between an intervention group (osteopathic treatment) and a control group (placebo treatment) after a step test in terms of RPD (Rating of Perceived Dyspnoea) dyspnoea perception during exercise.

CHAPTER 7

Method

The following section lists how the author addressed the question of what effect or measurable impact osteopathy has on healthy adults.

7.1 Literature

In order to examine the topic as comprehensively as possible, a literature review was conducted between November 2014 and June 2015 on the Internet and in the libraries of the Medical University of Vienna and Danube University Krems.

The following table shows the relevant databases, journals and keywords used.

7.1.1 Databases, journals, keywords

Databases	• Sciencedirect • Osteopathy Research • Pedro • Physio Pedia • Google Scholar • Cochrane Library • PubMed • Medpilot
Journals	• Journal of Bodywork and Movement Therapies • European Respiratory Journal • American Journal of Respiratory and Critical Care Medicine • Osteopathic Medicine • International Journal of Osteopathic Medicine
Keywords	• Osteopathy • Spirometry • Effectiveness • Borg Scale/CR10 • Cardiopulmonary exercise tests • Respiratory dysfunction • Diaphragm • Prevention
	• Somatic dysfunction • Placebo/sham treatment • Health promotion • Respiratory system • Respiratory mechanics

7.2 Study design

This experimental randomised controlled clinical study was conducted using a between-subject design (intervention and placebo group).

The osteopathic treatments in the intervention group were performed by an osteopath with five years of professional experience. The examination and treatment results were documented (see Appendix A).

The control group participated in a placebo or sham treatment (inactive microwave).

The students involved had not yet attended any courses on this aspect of electrophysical therapy and therefore had no expectations regarding microwave therapy. This measure was carried out by a physiotherapist with 10 years of professional experience ( ).

7.3 Sample description

This section provides a tabular overview of the inclusion and exclusion criteria for the group of people examined.

7.3.1 Inclusion criteria

Table 3 Inclusion criteria

• Healthy men and women aged between 18 and 38
• Students in their second semester of a physiotherapy degree programme at the IMC University of Applied Sciences Krems.
• Signing of a form agreeing to participate in this study on a voluntary basis.

7.3.2 Exclusion criteria

Table 4 Exclusion criteria

• Acute fractures
• Acute infections
• Pregnancy
• Current use of painkillers or anti-inflammatory medication
• Significant psychological or emotional stress

7.3.3 Sample size and sampling

A total of 24 female test subjects were recruited for participation. All of them were included in the study. To ensure that the test subjects were familiar with the spirometry tests and the modified Borg scale for self-assessment, the spirometry and the Borg scale were discussed and practised with each individual test subject in advance.

The baseline data was collected after a three-minute step test using a spirometer and the BORG score.

This group was composed as follows:

Characteristics		Baseline	
		Test group	Control
n =		14	10
Age:		23.8 ±3.87	23.8 ±5.56
Gender	m	50	40
	f	50	60
Weight:	kg	68.14 ±12.31	64.1 ± 10.07
Size:	cm	173.9 ± 7.89	170.4 ±7.64

Figure 1 Baseline data (own representation)

7.4 Test materials

At this point, the test and assessment procedures used are listed and briefly explained and described, and the evidence base is briefly discussed.

7.4.1 Three-minute step test

In order to further homogenise the test subjects and to investigate the effect of osteopathy on changes in lung function under stress, a standardised cardiopulmonary stress test is performed. The 3-minute step test is suitable for this purpose.
This stress test was introduced as a cardiorespiratory stress test by Kasch and colleagues back in 1965 (Kasch FW., 1965). Despite weaknesses in reliability and validity (Kool J., 2011), this test is suitable as a general test of physical performance (Ritchie C., 2005). (Burnstein Bryan D., Reliability of Fitness Tests using methods and time periods common in sport and occupational management, 2011). It was particularly important to the author that this allowed the cardiorespiratory system to be transferred to a real stress situation. At the same time, it was also possible to document a subjective parameter afterwards. This modified BORG scale is now explained.

7.4.2 Modified Borg scale

The modified Borg scale is used to quantitatively record the subjective perception or perceived exertion of the participants in the experimental part of the study.
This CR-10 scale category ratio according to Borg is a widely used method and was developed from the Borg Rating of Perceived Exertion Scale. The numbers are accompanied by non-linear verbal descriptors. For example, the number 0 is assigned the description "not at all" for breathing effort, and the anchor point 10 is assigned the description "maximum". It can be used to determine all types of sensations, e.g. dyspnoea during physical exertion. It also shows good reproducibility in healthy individuals (Meyer FJ., 2013, p. 19).

7.4.3 Spirometer

A mobile spirometer (Gare Fusion Micro I) is used to objectify the examination described in the experimental section.
Spirometry is a simple, practical, non-invasive and inexpensive test for measuring lung volumes and respiratory flow rates (Criee C.-P., 2006, p. 1).
Miller aptly describes it as follows:

"Spirometry is a physiological test that measures how much air a person inhales and exhales over a period of time. The primary signal measured in spirometry can be volume or flow. Spirometry is as valuable a screening test for general respiratory health as blood pressure measurement is for general cardiovascular health" (Miller M.R, 2005, p. 320).

Miller describes a number of indications, including for public health, e.g. epidemiological surveys and clinical research (Miller M.R, 2005, p. 320).

The measurement parameters obtained are divided into static and dynamic lung volumes. Static lung volumes are lung volumes whose measured values do not depend on the time course of the spirogram, e.g. vital capacity (VC). Dynamic lung volumes include forced expiratory volume in one second (FEV1). The volume that can be exhaled after maximum inspiration by forced expiration in the first second is referred to as (absolute) forced expiratory volume in one second (FEV1) (Criee C.-P., 2006, p. 3-5).

7.5 Study procedure

Forty students in their second semester of a physiotherapy course were informed about the planned study at the beginning of February.

The students were informed about the procedure and voluntary participation and were allowed to participate if they met the inclusion criteria.

The examinations and tests were carried out between 3 March and 25 March 2015 on the premises of the IMC FH Krems Campus West.

The initial examinations were completed on 13 March.

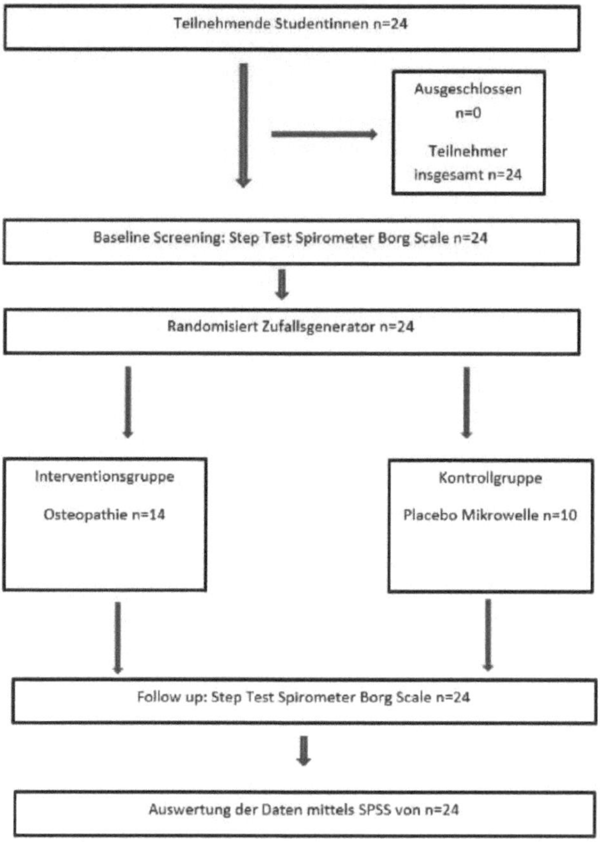

Figure 2: Flowchart of the study procedure (own representation)

7. Data processing and analysis

The tables and figures were created using Windows Excel and Word.

The statistical data was evaluated and graphically represented using the statistical programme Microsoft

SPSS Version 20.

CHAPTER 8

Results

The results are presented and briefly described in the following section in the form of figures and tables.

8.1 Baseline data

Characteristics		Baseline		Follow-up	
		Test group	control group	Experimental group	Control group
n =		14	10	14	10
Age:		23.8 ±3.87	23.8 ±5.56	23.8 ±3.87	23.8 ±5.56
Gender:	m	50	40	50	40
	w	50	60	50	60
Weight:		68.14 ±12.31	64.1 ±10.07	68.14 ±12.31	64.1 ±10.07
Size:	cm	173.9 ±7.89	170.4 ±7.64	173.9 ±7.89	170.4 ±7.64
FEV 1 (mean+ SD):		4.16 ±0.85	3.77 ±0.6	4.05 ± 0.82	3.7 ±0.57
RPE (mean+ SD):		12.21 ±2.2	11.9 ± 2.02	11.85 ±2.26	12.0 ±1.55
RPD (mean + SD):		12.14 ±1.52	11.8 ±1.78	11.5 ± 1.49	11.7 ±1.61

Figure 3 Demographic data baseline and follow-up (own representation)

The median values of the demographic data were evaluated and a descriptive data analysis was performed for the differences in RPE (received perception of exertion), RPD (received perception of dyspnoea) and FEV1 (forced expiratory volume in the first second).

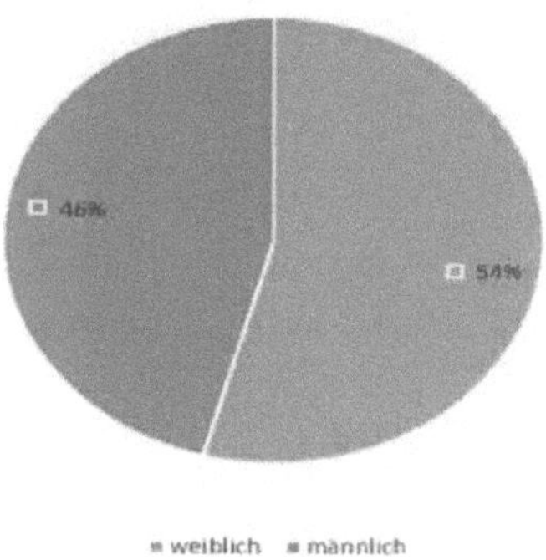

Figure 4: Gender distribution

This pie chart shows the distribution of the 24 test subjects into an approximately equal distribution of men (46% n=11) and women (54% n=13).

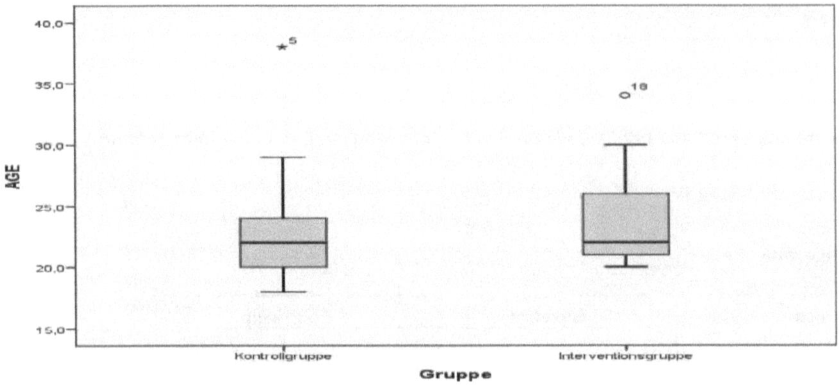

Figure 5: Age distribution of the group

This graph shows that the age distribution in both groups has a similar starting point.

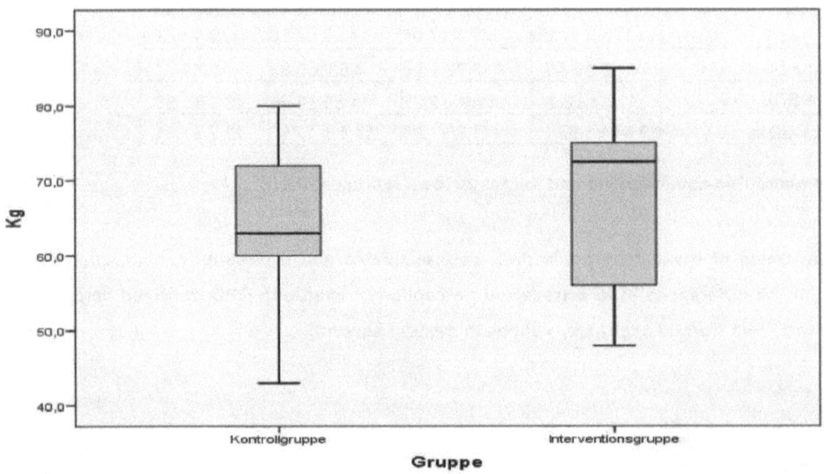

Figure 6: Weight distribution of the group

The following graph shows a similar starting point for both groups in terms of the median value (weight), but the standard deviations show that both groups have a wide range.

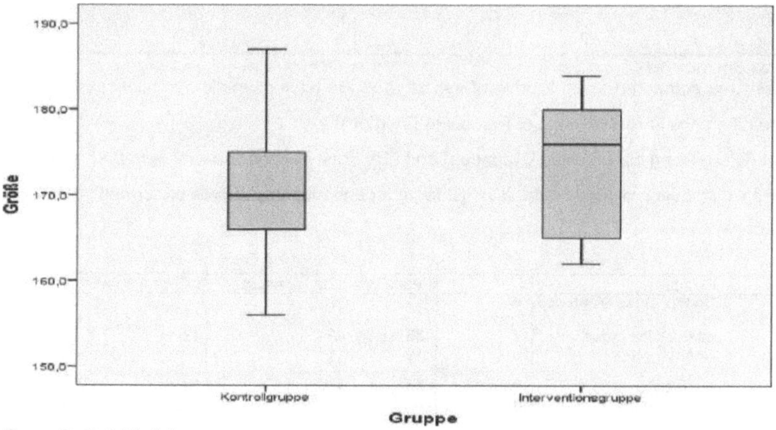

Figure 7: Height of the group

The following graph shows a similar starting point for both groups in terms of the median value (height), but the standard deviations indicate that both groups show a large variation.

8.2 Evaluation of the differences

In a further evaluation step, a descriptive data analysis was performed for the differences in RPE (Received Perception of Exertion) and RPD (Received Perception of Dyspnea) as well as for the FEV1 (forced expiratory volume in the first second) values.

	N	Mean	Std. deviation	Min	Max	Percentiles
						25th
Difference RPE	24	-.17	1.04	-	2	.00
RPD difference	24	-.42	1.06	-	2	-1.75
FEV1 L difference	24	-,08	.15	-.61	.14	-.15
Group	24	1.58	,50	1	2	1

	Percentiles	
	50th (median)	75th
Difference RPE	,	.00
RPD difference	.00	,00
FEV1 L difference	-,07	,020
Group	2	2

Figure 8 Descriptive statistics

In a second step, the normal distribution of the data was checked using the KS test. The results show that the difference values were not normally distributed in either the control group or the intervention group.

8.2.1 Two-sample Kolmogorov-Smirnov test

		Difference RPE	RPD difference	FEV1 L difference
Most Extreme Differences	Absolute	,	.20	0.27
	Positive	,30	,20	,27
	Negative	-.05	.00	-.07

Kolmogorov-Smirnov Z	.72	.48	.65
Asymp. Sig. (2-tailed)	.67	.97	.78

Figure 9 Kolmogorov Smirnov test

The significance test was compared using a table of values, and the asymptomatic significance showed a value of 0.67 for the difference in RPE (Rating of Perceived Exertion).

The other values for RPD (Rating of Perceived Dyspnoea) and FEV1 one-second capacity were 0.97 and 0.78.

Due to the non-normal distribution of these data, a T-test for independent samples was performed.

8.3 T-test

	Group	N	Mean	Std. deviation	Std. error Mean
RPE	Control group Difference	10	.	1	0
	Intervention group	14	-,36	.74	,19
RPD difference	Control group	10	-,10	1	,
	Intervention group	14	-,64	.92	,24
FEV1 L difference	Control group	10	-,06	,12	0.038
	Intervention group	14	-,11	.17	0.046

Figure 10 T-test

A confidence interval of 95% was assumed for the assessment of the significance level. Using the Leven test, it was determined that all variances in the evaluation are equal.

This results in a significance for the difference in RPE of p=0.30 in the T-test,

for the difference in RPD of p=0.22 and for the difference in Fev1 of p=0.43.

8.4 Leven test

Independent Samples Test

		Levene's test for equality of variances		I-test Equality of Means						
									95%Mdeo Internall ofthe Difference	
		.	Sig.	t	df	Sig. (2-tailed)	Nean Differente	Std.Efror Difference	Lower	Upper
Dilf&renzRP E	Equivariances assumed	1.694	,207	1.055	22	,303	,457	.433	-.412	1,356
	Equal variances not assumed			.959	12.806	.356	.457	.477	-,575	1,499
RPD difference	Equivariances assumed	0.065	0.802	1.252	2	.224	,543	,433	-,356	1,442
	Equal variances not assumed			1.199	16.314	.248	.543	.453	-.415	1,501
FEVILDiffeierz	Equal variances assumed	.161	.692	.789	22	.439	.05071	.06428	-,08260	,18403
	Equal variances not assumed			,837	22,000	,411	.05071	0.06058	.07492	.17635

Figure 11: Leven test

8.5 Summary of hypotheses

Null hypothesis HO

There is no difference between an intervention group (osteopathic treatment) and a control group (placebo treatment) after a step test in terms of the lung function value FEV1.

Based on the evaluation of the T-test and the result of p=0.43, the null hypothesis must be accepted.

Secondary hypothesis 02

There is no difference between an intervention group (osteopathic treatment) and a control group (placebo treatment) in terms of the RPE (Rating of Perceived Exertion) of the test subjects' cardiopulmonary exertion.
Based on the evaluation of the T-test and the result of $p=0.30$, secondary hypothesis 02 must be accepted.

Sub-hypothesis 03

There is no difference between an intervention group (osteopathic treatment) and a control group (placebo treatment) in terms of RPD (Rating of Perceived Dyspnoea) dyspnoea perception during exercise.
Based on the evaluation of the T-test and the result of $p=0.22$, secondary hypothesis 03 must be accepted.

CHAPTER 9

Discussion

In this section, the present pilot study will be analysed and reflected upon once again. The aim is to carry out an error analysis of all areas and to consider possible ways of continuing this idea.
To this end, all chapters and their respective subcategories will be discussed individually.

9.

The question of the optimal method, or whether randomised controlled trials are the best way to research osteopathy and its effects on humans, is still the subject of heated debate in the scientific community.
Perhaps other designs, such as pragmatic designs, should be given more weight, and the cohort studied, the patients and contextual factors should also be given greater consideration (Leach, 2008).
This often involves the problem that attempts to achieve too high internal validity often impair transferability to reality in terms of external validity (Milanese, 2011).
Future generations of osteopaths should continue to be inspired by AT Still, who was able to combine science and holism at the very beginning of osteopathy (Leach, 2008).

Patient collective

The opportunity to recruit a healthy group of test subjects through our own workplace at the IMC FH Krems Physiotherapy programme was a valuable experience.
This gave students the opportunity to participate in a real-life project.
The following table has already been used in the results. For a better overview, it is reproduced here to clearly present all data for discussion.

Characteristics		**Baseline**		**Follow-up**	
		Experimental group	Control group	Experimental group	Control group
n =		14	10	14	10
Age:		23.3	23.8± 5.56	23.8 ±3.87	23.8 ±5.56
Gender:	m	50	40	50	40
	w	50	60	50	60
Weight:		68.14 ±12.31	64.1 ±10.07	68.14 ± 12.31	64.1 ± 10.07
Height:	cm	173.9 ±7.89	170.4 ± 7.64	173.9 ±7.39	170.4 ± 7.64
FEV 1 (mean + SD):		4.16 ±0.85	3.77±0.6	4.05 ± 0.82	3.7 ±0.57
RPE (mean + SD):		12.21 ±2.2	11.9 ±2.02	11.85 ±2.26	12.0 ± 1.55
RPD (mean + SD):		12.14 ±1.52	11.8 ±1.78	11.5 ±1.49	11.7 ±1.61

Figure 12 Discussion Demographic data baseline and follow-up

The test group represents a healthy group of young people who showed the following median values: age (intervention group) ~24 years, height 1.74 cm, and weight - 68 kg. This weight corresponds to a BMI (body mass index) of 23. This BMI is interpreted as normal body weight (WHO, Global Database on Body Mass Index, 2015).
The ratio of men to women (intervention group) was almost 50:50.
The baseline values for the FEV1 spirometry measurement were above average despite a three-minute step

test performed beforehand. This reduced the sensitivity of the test, as this lung parameter was already at an excellent level.

The table below shows the average demographic values with standard values for FEV1 reference values for the relevant age group for men (Ebinger, 2015) (Haber & Popovic, Pumopret, 2015).

Table 5: Median baseline values and standard values (own representation)

Age (years)	**Height** (cm)	**Weight** (kg)	**Blood pressure** (mmHG)	**Baseline** FEV1	**Follow-up** FEV1	**Normal value** FEV1
-24	**-174**	**-68**	**760**	**4.16**	**4.05**	**4.3-4.54**

The average rating on the BORG RPE (Rating of Perceived Exertion) scale was ~12 (corresponding to "easy") and on the modified BORG RPD (Rating of Perceived Dyspnoea) scale was also ~12 (corresponding to "low").

Here too, the group performed very well, indicating a healthy cardiovascular system.

Literature review

The literature review was not sufficiently critical. When selecting randomised controlled trials in various databases, for example, the Pedro scale or the Delphi list should have been used. This creates better conditions for easily recognising whether the available RCTs are internally valid and contain sufficient statistical information to make the results interpretable (Hegenscheidt & Harth, 2015).

9.2

The statistical analysis showed that the null hypothesis HO, i.e. there is no difference between an intervention group (osteopathic treatment) and a control group (placebo treatment) after a step test in terms of the lung function value FEV1, must be accepted with a p-value of 0.43 based on the T-test performed afterwards. This result should not be overestimated, however, because, as already listed in the chapter "Study situation and measures", some authors have already been able to demonstrate positive effects on lung capacity in healthy and sick individuals through individual manual techniques and through standardisation of an osteopathic treatment procedure.

The author was aware before the start of the study that the objective parameters might not be sufficiently clear. Therefore, secondary hypotheses were also formulated. These were primarily intended to capture fluctuations in the subjective parameters collected.

Sub-hypothesis 02 states that there is no difference between an intervention group (osteopathic treatment) and a control group (placebo treatment) in terms of RPE (Rating of Perceived Exertion) of the test subjects' cardiopulmonary exertion, and with a value of p=0.30, sub-hypothesis 02 must be accepted.

Similarly, for secondary hypothesis 03, there is no difference between an intervention group (osteopathic treatment) and a control group (placebo treatment) in terms of RPD (Rating of Perceived Dyspnoea) dyspnoea perception during exercise, and with a value of p=0.22, secondary hypothesis 03 must also be accepted.

These results indicate that the modified BORG scale may not be sufficiently sensitive for these purposes.

Osteopathic intervention

During the osteopathic examination and treatment, it was noticed that the subjects were not homogeneous from an osteopathic point of view. This means that the number of identified somatic dysfunctions varied considerably (see the open box of findings in Appendix A).

Further subclassification could remedy this. Only then should the subjects be randomised into a treatment group and a control group with, for example, a similar number or similar types of dysfunctions according to osteopathic diagnosis in order to increase internal validity. Subjects with few or no dysfunctions are excluded from the study.

This approach naturally requires a large number of subjects and is therefore difficult to implement in the context of a master's thesis by a single researcher. However, it could lead to more comprehensible results.

CHAPTER 10

Conclusion

Summary

Within the scope of this master's thesis, an experimental randomised controlled between-subject design (intervention and placebo group) with a total of 24 participants was used to investigate whether osteopathic treatment can alter subjective physical performance and lung function in healthy adults.

In order to satisfactorily address this question from an osteopathic perspective, the theoretical part of the thesis discussed prevention and health promotion and explained the traditional principles, the model of somatic dysfunction and the structure-function models, as well as clinical reasoning strategies.

The respiratory system and respiratory pattern dysfunction were explained and the viscero-fascial connections were described.

These focal points arose from the author's particular interest in breathing pattern dysfunction and the effect of osteopathy on the respiratory system.

Breathing pattern dysfunction is often overlooked or not given sufficient importance.

This paper aims to investigate the extent to which the respiratory system can be influenced by osteopathic treatment prior to physical activity such as the step test. To objectify these effects, a spirometer and a BORG or modified BORG scale were used.

10.1 Conclusion

The research question posed: Can osteopathic treatment immediately change subjective physical performance and lung function in healthy adults? This question cannot yet be answered satisfactorily.

The data obtained show that osteopathy is not superior to placebo treatment.

This result, which was surprising to the author, should not be overestimated due to a number of errors.

The selection of more optimal assessment tools, the associated reduction of measurement errors and the testing of a larger cohort are necessary in order to arrive at a clearer statement.

As a suggestion for further studies of this kind, more complex measurement methods such as whole-body plethysmography (large lung function) could be used, which offer greater measurement accuracy and allow additional lung volumes to be determined.

Chaitow (Chaitow Leon, 2002, pp. 207-212) and McLaughlin (McLaughlin, 2009) have had good experience with capnometry (determination of carbon dioxide in exhaled air) in their studies to observe the optimal function of the respiratory system.

Blood gas analysis would also be a suitable, albeit more invasive, method of providing information about the distribution of oxygen and carbon dioxide gases and the pH value of the test subjects.

10.2 Outlook

Since prevention and health promotion are necessary strategies for ensuring that the healthcare system remains financially viable in the future, osteopathy should secure a permanent place in this field.

To this end, the number of RCT studies with an osteopathic perspective must be significantly increased in order to satisfactorily answer the question of osteopathy's effect on the respiratory system.

Osteopathic research must continue to look for suitable and sensitive assessment tools that can substantiate the effect of osteopathy in this area.

Finally, it should be noted that osteopathy, with its subtle manual examination and treatment approaches, is a valuable option for detecting and treating physical dysfunctions at an early stage.

The intensive personal and physical attention given to patients should be emphasised, as this is increasingly neglected in a technologised society under constant time and performance pressure.

Bibliography

(25 March 2015). Retrieved from Pubmed.de: http://www.pubmed.de/no_cache/zufallsgenerator/

AAOM. (18 December 2011). *American Association of Colleges of Osteopathic Medicine.* Retrieved from Glossary: www.aacom.org

Associations, E. F. (8 March 2015). *European Federation of Allergy and Airways Diseases Patients' Associations (EFA).* Retrieved from http://www.efanet.org/diseases-allergies/abgerufen

Batrow, K. (2012). *Examination and Diagnosis in Physiotherapy.* Würzburg: Springer.

Biberschick, M. (1 May 2015). *Osteopathic Research Web.* Retrieved from http://www.osteopathic-research.com/index.php?option=com_jresearch&view=publication&task=show&id=14311&lang=en

Böhmüller, E. (08. 05 2007). *The influence of an osteopathic treatment on the performance of a high-performance athlete.* Retrieved from www.osteopathicresearch.com: www.osteopathicresearch.com/paper_pdf/BoehmuellerElke.pdf

Bortz, W. (2011). *Next Medicine: The science and civics of health.* Oxford: Oxford University Press.

Bradley, D. (2002). Patterns of breathing dysfunction in hyperventilation syndrome and breathing pattern disorders. In L. Chaitow, D. Bradley, & C. Gilbert, *Multidisciplinary approaches to breathing pattern disorders* (pp. 43-60). Edinburgh: Churchill Livingstone.

Bradley, H., & Esformes, J. (9 2014). Breathing pattern disorders and functional movement. *Int. J.Sport Phys. Ther.,* pp. 28-39.

Buckup, K. (2009). *Clinical tests on bones, joints and muscles.* Stuttgart: Thieme.

Burnstein Bryan D., S. R. (5 October 2011). Reliability of fitness tests using methods and time periods common in sport and occupational management. *Journal of Athletic Training,* pp. 505–513.

Burnstein Bryan D., S. R. (5 October 2011). Reliability of fitness tests using methods and time periods common in sport and occupational management. *Journal of Athletic Training,* pp. 505–513.

Chaitow Leon, B. D. (2002). *Multidisciplinary approaches to breathing pattern disorders.* Edinburgh: Churchill Livingstone.

Chaitow, L. (7 2004). Breathing pattern disorders, motor control, and low back pain. *Journal of Osteopathic Medicine,* pp. 33-40.

Chaitow, L. (03. 05 2015). *Physiopedia.* From http://www.physio-pedia.eom/Breathing_Pattern_Disorders#cite_ref-Lum_0-0 accessed

Chaitow, L., Gilbert, C., & Lovegrov, J. (2012). Breathing and chronic pelvic pain: Connections and rehabilitation features. In L. Chaitow, & R. Lovegrove Jones, *Chronic pelvic pain and dysfunction; Practical Physical Medicine* (pp. 193-226). Churchill Livingston Elsevier.

Chin, L. M., Leigh, R. J., Heigenhauser, G. J., Rossiter, H. B., Paterson, D. H., & Kowalchuk, J. M. (15 August 2007). Hyperventilation-induced hypocapnic alkalosis slows the adaptation of pulmonary 02 uptake during the transition to moderate-intensity exercise. *The Journal of Physiology,* pp. 351-364.

Corts, M. (2012). *Diagnostic guide to osteopathy.* Stuttgart: Haug.

Courtney, R. (12 December 2009). The function of breathing and its dysfunction and their relationship to breathing therapy. *International Journal of Osteopathic Medicine,* pp. 78–85.

Criee C.-P., B. D. (2006). *German Respiratory League.* Retrieved from the German Society for Pneumology:www.atemwegsliga.de/empfehlungen-positionspapiere.html Dennison, L. (8 April 2015). A *Quantitative Experiment to Assess the Effects of Osteopathic Treatment Targeting the Diaphragm on Chest Wall Mobility.* Retrieved from The British School of Osteopathy: http://opac.bso.ac.uk

DL, S. (2000). *Evidence-based medicine: how to practice and teach EBM.* Edinburgh: Churchill Livingston.

Donald R. Noll, D., Brian F. Degenhardt, D., Christian Fossum, D. (., & Kendi Hensel, D. (09 2008). Clinical and Research Protocol for Osteopathic Manipulative Treatment of Elderly Patients With Pneumonia. *JAOA,* pp. 508-516.

Donald R. Noll, D., Brian F. Degenhardt, D., Jane C. Johnson, M., & Selina A. Burt, D. (05 2008). Immediate Effects of Osteopathic Manipulative Treatment in Elderly Patients With Chronic Obstructive Pulmonary Disease. *JAOA,* pp. 251-259.

e.V., B. f. (22 May 2015). *Professional Association for Osteopathic Medicine, hpO.* Retrieved from http://www.hpo-osteopathie.de/aktuelles_presse

Ebinger, A. (15 May 2015). *Easier breathing.* Retrieved from http://www.leichter-atmen.de/lexikon-fev1

Farthing, R., Gosling, C., Williams, K., & Vaughan, B. (9 2006). The effect of different rates of application of rib raising technique on cardiovascular and respiratory measures in asymptomatic individuals. *International Journal of Osteopathic Medicine,* pp. 27-46.

Finet, G., & Williame, C. (2012). *Visceral Osteopathy.* Mons: Self-published.

Fink-Koller, B. (20 May 2015). *Osteopathic Research.* Retrieved from http://www.osteopathic- research.com: http://www.osteopathic-research.com/paper_pdf/Fink-KollerBirgit.pdf

Fossum, C. (10 May 2015). *Osteopathic European Academic Network.* Retrieved from http://www.osean.com/index.php/resources/doc/doc_download/306-christian-fossum- osteopathic-education-and-research-from-apprenticeship-to-information-mastery

Francisco Jose Gonzales-Alvarez, M. C.-M.-S.-D. (08 2014). *Effects of diaphragm stretching technique on pulmonary function in healthy participants: A randomised-controlled trial.*
From

Froom, P., & Benbassat, J. (2000). Inconsistencies in the Classification of Preventive Interventions. *Preventive Medicine 31,* pp. 153-158.

Health, B. f. (5 May 2015). *Federal Ministry of Health.* Retrieved from http://www.bmg.gv.at/cms/home/attachments/3/4/4/CH1066/CMS1291414949078/ge sundheitssystem-zahlen-daten-2013.pdf

Gibbons, T. (2004). *Manipulation of the Spine, Thorax and Pelvis: Osteopathic Diagnosis and Therapy.*

Munich: Elsevier.

Goyal, S. (10 May 2015). *An Experiment to Assess the Effects of Osteopathic Treatment to the Diaphragm and Intercostal Muscles to Improve Oxygen Saturation Levels in Healthy Volunteers.* From The British School of Osteopathy: http://opac.bso.ac.uk accessed

Greenman, P. E. (1998). *Textbook of Osteopathic Medicine.* Heidelberg: Haug.

Haber, P., & Popovic, R. (15 May 2015). *Pulmopret.* Retrieved from http://www.pulmopret.at/online

Haber, P., & Popovic, R. (15 May 2015). *Pumopret.* Retrieved from http://www.pulmopret.at/online

Hannah Lougee, M. G. (2013). The suitability of sham treatments for use as placebo control in trials of spinal manipulative therapy: A pilot study. *Journal of Bodywork and Movement Therapies,* pp. 59-68.

Hebgen, E. (2008). *Visceral osteopathy – fundamentals and techniques.* Stuttgart: Hippokrates. Hegenscheidt, S., & Harth, A. (01. 05 2015). *PEDro Physiotherapy Evidence Database.* Retrieved from http://www.pedro.org.au/german/downloads/pedro-scale/

Hellich, W. (05 2011). The immediate influence of osteopathy on the respiratory performance of members of the fire brigade.

Hellich, W. (May 2011). The immediate impact on the breathing performance of members of the fire brigade.

Hinkeltheim, E., & Zalpour, C. (2006). *Diagnostic and therapeutic concepts in osteopathy.* Heidelberg: Spinger Medizin Verlag.

Hofmarsch, M. M., & Rack, H. M. (07. 05 2015). *World Health Organisation Regional Office Europe.* From http://www.euro.who.int/___

Ismail-Tsaous, E. (2 February 2014). Subsidies for osteopathic treatments: benefits for insured persons and health insurance funds. *Osteopathic Medicine,* pp. 26–28.

Kasch FW., P. W. (4 May 1965). Maximum work capacity in middle-aged males by a step test method. *J Sports Med Phys Fitness,* pp. 198-202.

Key, J. e. (2 December 2007). A model of movement dysfunction provides a classification system guiding diagnosis and therapeutic care in spinal pain and related musculoskeletal syndromes: a paradigm shift. *Journal of Bodywork and Movement Therapies,* pp. 105–120.

Kimberly G Fulda, T. S. (12 January 2007). Patient expectations for placebo treatments commonly used in *osteopathic medicine and primary care. Osteopathic Medicine and Primary Care 1:3.*

Klaus, H., Theodor, K., & Jochen, H. (17 May 2014). Introduction: Disease prevention and health promotion. In H. Klaus, K. Theodor, & H. Jochen, *Textbook on Prevention and Health Promotion* (pp. 13-23). Bern: Huber. Retrieved from http://www.uni-ulm.de/fileadmin/website_uni_ulm/med.inst.020/Einf%C3%BChrungsscript_ab_SS_2 010.pdf accessed

Knieps, F. (03. 05 2015). *BKK umbrella organisation.* Retrieved from http://www.bkk-dachverband.de/fileadmin/publikationen/gesundheitsreport_2014/BKK_Gesundheitsr eport.pdf accessed

Kool J., O. P. (2011). Cardiopulmonary fitness: 3-minute step test. In H. R.-A. Oesch P., *Assessments in Rehabilitation* (pp. 206-208). Bern: Hans Huber.

Kuchera, M. L., & Kuchera, W. A. (1994). *Osteopathic Considerations in Systemic Dysfunction.* Columbus: Greyden Press.

Kuchera, W. A., & Kuchera, M. L. (1994). *Osteopathic Principles in Practice.* Columbo: Greyden Press.

Leach, J. (03 2008). I.Towards an osteopathic understanding of evidence. *International Journal of Osteopathic Medicine Volume 11; Issue 1,* pp. 3-6.

Liem, T. (2008). Developmental dynamics and holistic principles and their significance for osteopathy. In T. Liem, P. Sommerfeld, & P. Wührl, *Theories of Osteopathic Thinking and Action* (pp. 7-28). Stuttgart: Hippokrates.

McLaughlin, L. (11 January 2009). Breathing evaluation and retraining. *Journal of Bodywork and Movement Therapies 13,* pp. 276–282.

Meyer FJ., B. M.-B. (2013). Stress testing in pneumology Recommendation of the German Society for Pneumology and Respiratory Medicine *Pneumology,* pp. 16-34.

Milanese, S. (10 February 2011). The use of RCTs in manual therapy – Are we trying to fit a round peg into a square hole? *Manual Therapy 16,* pp. 403–405.

Miller M.R, H. J. (05. 04 2005). Standardisation of spirometry. *Eur Respir J,* pp. 319-338.

Nagel, M. (2008). Expert panel: Osteopathy in motion. In T. Liem, P. Sommerfeld, & P. Wührl, *Theories of osteopathic thinking and action* (pp. 131-149). Stuttgart: Hippokrates.

Osborn, G. G., & Jerome, J. A. (2011). Health Promotion and Maintenance. In A. G. Chila, *Foundations of Osteopathic Medicine* (pp. 377-386). Philadelphia: Lippincott; Williams & Wilkins.

Osteopathy, A. A. (18 December 2011). *American Association of Colleges of Osteopathic Medicine.* Retrieved from Glossary: www.aacom.org

P. Thompson, O. (16 March 2013). *International Journal of Osteopathic Medicine,* pp. 25-32.

Parson, J. (2006). *Osteopathy: Models for Diagnosis, Treatment and Practice.* Tottenham: Elservier.

Peper, E., & Tibbetts, V. (10 May 2015). *Biofeedback Federation of Europe.* Retrieved from http://bfe.org/articles/M%FChelose%20Zwerchfell%20Atmung.pdf

Rauch, A. (2012). Methodology (introduction, basics, concept). Lecture notes, Vienna School of Osteopathy.

Richter, P., & Hebgen, E. (2007). *Trigger Points and Muscle Function Chains.* Stuttgart: Hippokrates.

Risch, A. J. (05. 04 2015). *Osteoapathic Research Web.* Retrieved from http://www.osteopathic-research.com/index.php?option=com_jresearch&view=publication&task=show&id=14976&lang=en

Ritchie C., T. S. (1 August 2005). Reliability and validity of physical fitness field test for adults aged 55 to 70 years. *J Sci Med Sport,* pp. 61-70.

Rosenbrock, R., & Gerlinger, T. (2006). *Health Policy: A Systemic Introduction.* Bern: Huber.

Sackett DL, R. W. (Sackett DL, Rosenberg WMC, Gray JAM, Haynes RB, Richardson WS. Evidence-based Medicine: What It Is and What It Isn't. In: British Medical Journal. 312, 1996, pp. 71-72. 1996). What It Is and What It Isn't. *British Medical Journal,* pp. 71-72.

Seffinger, M. A., King, H. H., Ward, R. C., Jones, J. M., Rogers, F. J., & Patterson, M. M. (2011). Osteopathy Philosophy. In A. G. Chila, *Foundation of Osteopathic Medicine Third Edition* (pp. 3-22). Baltimore: Lippincott Williams & Wilkins.

Sidler, S. (03 2010). The relevance of intuition in osteopathy – considerations and a literature review. *Osteopathic Medicine, Journal for Holistic Healing Methods,* pp. 4–9.

Stark, J. (2007). *Still's Fascial Concepts.* Jolandos.

Steinbach, H. (2007). Health promotion: A textbook for nursing and healthcare professions. In H. Steinbach, *Health promotion: A textbook for nursing and healthcare professions* (p. 43). Vienna: Facultas.

Stone, C. (2002). *Science in the Art of Osteopathy: Osteopathic Principles and Practice.* Cheltenham: Nelson Thornes Ltd.

Swonar, B. (03. 04 2015). *Medical University of Graz.* Retrieved from http://public-health.medunigraz.at/archiv/Mastersarbeiten/Masterarbeit_10/Abstract_MT_BrigitteS wonar.pdf

Thomas, M., McKinley, R., Freeman, E., & Foy, C. (14 April 2005). The prevalence of dysfunctional breathing in adults in the community with and without asthma. *Prim Care Respir J.,* pp. 78-82.

Thomson, O. P., Petty, N. J., & Moore, A. P. (06 2011). Clinical reasoning in osteopathy - More than just principles? *International Journal of Osteopathic Medicine Volume 14 Issue 2,* pp. 71-76.

Thomson, O. P., Petty, N. J., & Moore, A. P. (06 2014). Diagnostic reasoning in osteopathy- A qualitative study. *International Journal of Osteopathic Medicine Volume 12, Issue 2, pp.* 83-93.

Tilscher, U. P. (01. 05 2015). *Responsible prevention.* Retrieved from http://www.responsible- prevention.com/

Vielitz, A. (01. 05 2015). *Screening questionnaire.* Retrieved from http://screeningbogen.de/zipt_screeningbogen.pdf

Ward, R. (2003). *Foundations for Osteopathic Medicine, Mission Statement.* Lippincott Williams & Wilkins.

Wheatley, A., Gosling, C., & Gibbons, P. (3 2000). Investigation of the effects of using a rib raising technique on FEV1 and FVC outcomes in people with asthma: a clinical investigation. *Journal of Osteopathic Medicine,* pp. 60-64.

WHO. (1946). Constitution. Geneva: WHO.

WHO. (1986). Ottawa Charter. Ottawa: WHO.

WHO. (14 December 2014). *The Forum for Osteopathic Regulation in Europe.* Retrieved from http://www.forewards.eu/app/download/5219416/WHO+Benchmarks.pdf

WHO. (15 05 2015). *Global Database on Body Mass Index.* Retrieved from http://apps.who.int/bmi/index.jsp?introPage=intro_3.html

Wikipedia. (10. 05 2015). *Wikipedia The free encyclopaedia.* From http://de.wikipedia.Org/wiki/Hypokapnie#cite_note-1

Wikipedia. (18. 05 2015). *Wikipedia The free encyclopaedia.* From http://de.wikipedia.org/wiki/Intuition accessed

Willard, F. H. (2011). Mechanics of Respiration. In A. G. Chila, *Foundations of Osteopathic Medicine, third edition* (pp. 207-220). Philadelphia: Lippincott Williams & Wilkins.

Zalpour, C. (2006). *Anatomy and Physiotherapy for Physiotherapy.* Munich: Elservier.

Appendix A

Self-assessment questionnaire / spirometer data sheet Baseline

First name ______ (initials) Surname __________________ Date ______________ 2015

Age ________ (years) Gender ____________________ (M/F)

Weight: __________(kg) Origin ______________ (European/non-European/Asian/other)

RPERPD	Perceived exertion	Dyspnoea
6		
7	Very very slight	none
8		
9	very easy	hardly
10		
11	easy	low
12		
13	Somewhat strenuous	considerable
14		
15	exhausting	very
16		
17	very difficult	very strong
18		
19	very very severe	very very strong
20	too strong, no longer possible	

Spirometer

Basic	Best breath of 3	%Prog
FEV1		
FVC		
FEV1/FVC		
PEF		

Self-assessment form / spirometer data sheet Follow-up

First name____(initials) Surname____ Date_____ 2015

Alter______(Jahre) Geschlecht______(M/W)

Weight:_____(kg) Origin______(European/non-European/Asian/other)

RPERPD	Perceived exertion	Dyspnoea
6		
7	Very very slight	none
8		
9	very easy	hardly
10		
11	easy	low
12		
13	Somewhat strenuous	considerable
14		
15	exhausting	very
16		
17	very difficult	very strong
18		
19	very very severe	very very strong
20	too strong, no longer possible	

Spirometer

Basic	Best of 3 breaths	%Prog
FEV1		
FVC		
FEV1/FVC		
PEF		

Medical history form

Dear Sir or Madam,

This form is intended to ensure safe osteopathic treatment and to rule out other causes of your symptoms. The more your osteopath knows about your health, the safer and more effective the treatment will be.

Please try to answer all questions as best you can.

If you are unable or unwilling to answer a question, please mark it with a question mark.

Any open questions will be discussed during the treatment.

Your information is subject to therapeutic confidentiality.

Name First name Date

Age Height Weight: Gender

1. Question: Are you currently feeling generally unwell or ill?
2. Question: Do you have a fever or elevated temperature?
3. Question: Are you under medical treatment?
4. Question: How long have you had these symptoms?
5. Question: Have your symptoms worsened significantly in the last two weeks?
6. Question: Are your symptoms caused by an event or injury?
7. Question: Do you have constant pain?
8. Question: Do you also experience pain when resting?
9. Question: Do you have pain at night?
10. Question: Are your symptoms independent of movement and/or posture?
11. Question: Is there any movement that you are no longer able to perform?
12. Question: Do you experience any of the following symptoms?

    Tingling: Numbness: Paralysis: Spasticity

13. Question: Please rate your maximum pain level over the last 24 hours on a scale of 0-10.

    24 hours

14. Question: Have you been diagnosed with heart problems?
15. Question: Do you experience chest pain during periods of physical exertion?
16. Question: Do you know of any possible reasons why you are unable to engage in physical exertion?

17. Question: Do you have any illnesses or conditions such as:

diabetes, osteoporosis, cancer, arteriosclerosis, hepatitis, HIV, tuberculosis, organ disorders, glandular disorders, hormonal disorders, blood

Coagulation disorders Neurological diseases

18. Question: Are you taking any medication or hormones?
19. Question: Have you ever had any broken bones or operations?
20. Question: Do you suffer from frequent infections?
21. Question: Have you lost weight unintentionally in the last few months?
22. Question: Are you addicted to drugs, alcohol or medication?
23. Question: Do you suffer from headaches?
24. Question: Do you suffer from dizziness, nausea or vomiting?
25. Question: Do you have balance problems or do you sometimes fall?
26. Question: Do you sometimes lose consciousness?
27. Question: Do you sometimes involuntarily lose control of your bladder or bowel movements?
28. Question: Do you experience loss of strength in your arms or legs?

The following screening questionnaire was approved after consultation with the authors
(Vielitz, 2015)

Declaration of consent

Name of the patient in block letters.
Date of birth: ....
Code ....

I agree to participate in this clinical study.
With the following question:

Can osteopathic treatment change the subjective physical capacity and lung function of healthy adults?

Mr Pichler has provided me with detailed and comprehensible verbal information about the inclusion and exclusion criteria and the aim and purpose of the study.
Any questions I had were answered clearly and satisfactorily by the osteopath.

I had sufficient time to make my decision.
I will comply with the instructions necessary for the conduct of the clinical study, but reserve the right to terminate my voluntary participation at any time without incurring any disadvantages.
I agree that the data collected about me in the course of this clinical trial may be recorded.
The provisions of the Data Protection Act will be observed when handling the data. I have received a copy of this patient information and consent form. The original will remain with the osteopath.

Date Signature of participants

Explanation of the following section: Findings form for osteopathic treatment

This part of the appendix contains the fourteen findings forms for the intervention group.
These forms were used for all participants. The findings that stood out, the somatic dysfunctions identified by the practitioner and the measures taken were recorded. These areas were marked with an ellipse symbol:

Findings form for osteopathic treatment Date Case 1

Medical history form was completed by each participant (see Appendix A Medical history form) No immediate contraindications for manual treatment could be identified. Gender: Male Age: 30 years Height: 170 cm Weight: 74 kg

Hypothesis 1: Does a 15-minute osteopathic treatment have an effect on lung function or on the subjective perception of exertion and dyspnoea?

Tick off standardised procedure after completion:

Findings:

Static and dynamic inspection Standing – sitting – supine

Special tests:

Provocation tests (complaint structure):

Palpation:

Oscillation test (somatic dysfunction of the spine, identification of segments):

Breathing movement test (number of breathing cycles, thoracic movement, diaphragm)

Intervention in the subsystems:

Craniosacral system

P.A.M

Rhythm Force Symmetry Amplitude

Visceral system

Subdiaphragmatic central lateral/left lateral right/right

Small pelvis

Parietal system

Cervical region: occiput, upper cervical spine, respiratory accessory muscles hypertonic

Thoracic region: clavicle, ribs and intercostal muscles, Th1-Th5, Th5-Th10; Th10-L2

Lumbosacral dysfunction

Pelvic congestion

Techniques:

Soft tissue techniques and fascial techniques

Muscle energy techniques and positional release techniques HVLA

Long lever techniques

Visceral techniques on the greater and lesser omentum and radix techniques, grand abdominal manoeuvre

Doming diaphragm

Rib raising

Cranial techniques

Findings form for osteopathic treatment Date Case 2

Medical history form was completed by each participant (see Appendix A Medical history form) No immediate contraindications to manual treatment could be identified. Gender: Male Age: 21 years Height: 180 cm Weight: 72 kg

Hypothesis 1: Does a 15-minute osteopathic treatment have an effect on lung function or on the subjective perception of exertion and dyspnoea?

Check off standardised procedure after completion:

Findings:

Static and dynamic inspection Standing – sitting – supine

Special tests:

Provocation tests (complaint structure):

Palpation:

Oscillation test (somatic dysfunction of the spine, identification of segments):

Breathing movement test (number of breathing cycles, thoracic movement, diaphragm)

Intervention in the subsystems:

Craniosacral system

P.A.M

Rhythm Force Symmetry Amplitude

Visceral system

Subdiaphragmatic central lateral/left lateral right/right

Small pelvis

Parietal system

Cervical region: occiput, upper cervical spine, respiratory accessory muscles hypertonic

Thoracic region: clavicle, ribs and intercostal muscles, Th1-Th5, Th5-Th10; Th10-L2

Lumbosacral dysfunction

Pelvic congestion

Techniques:

Soft tissue techniques and fascial techniques

Muscle energy techniques and positional release techniques HVLA

Long lever techniques

Visceral techniques on the greater and lesser omentum and radix techniques, grand abdominal manoeuvre

Doming diaphragm

Rib raising

Cranial techniques

Findings sheet for osteopathic treatment Date Case 3

Medical history form was completed by each participant (see Appendix A Medical history form) No immediate contraindications for manual treatment could be identified. Gender: Male Age: 23 years Height: 179 cm Weight: 73 kg

Hypothesis 1: Does a 15-minute osteopathic treatment have an effect on lung function or on the subjective perception of exertion and dyspnoea?

Check off standardised procedure after completion:

Findings:

Static and dynamic inspection Standing – sitting – supine position

Special tests:

Provocation tests (complaint structure):

Palpation:

Oscillation test (somatic dysfunction of the spine, identification of segments):

Breathing movement test (number of breathing cycles, thoracic movement, diaphragm)

Intervention in the subsystems:

Craniosacral system

P.A.M

Rhythm Force Symmetry Amplitude

Visceral system

Subdiaphragmatic central lateral/left lateral right/right

Small pelvis

Parietal system

Cervical region: occiput, upper cervical spine, respiratory accessory muscles hypertonic

Thoracic region: clavicle, ribs and intercostal muscles, Th1-Th5, Th5-Th10; Th10-L2

Lumbosacral dysfunction

Pelvic congestion

Techniques:

Soft tissue techniques and fascial techniques

Muscle energy techniques and positional release techniques HVLA

Long lever techniques

Visceral techniques on the greater and lesser omentum and radix techniques, grand abdominal manoeuvre

Doming diaphragm

Rib raising

Cranial techniques

Findings sheet for osteopathic treatment Date Case 4

Medical history form was completed by each participant (see Appendix A Medical history form) No immediate contraindications to manual treatment could be identified. Gender: Male Age: 22 years Height: 184 cm Weight: 83 kg

Hypothesis 1: Does a 15-minute osteopathic treatment have an effect on lung function or on the subjective perception of exertion and dyspnoea?

Check off standardised procedure after completion:

Findings:

Static and dynamic inspection Standing – sitting – supine

Special tests:

Provocation tests (complaint structure):

Palpation:

Oscillation test (somatic dysfunction of the spine, identification of segments):

Breathing movement test (number of breathing cycles, thoracic movement, diaphragm)

Intervention in the subsystems:

Craniosacral system

P.A.M

Rhythm Force Symmetry Amplitude

Visceral system

Subdiaphragmatic central lateral/left lateral right/right

Small pelvis

Parietal system

Cervical region: occiput, upper cervical spine, respiratory accessory muscles hypertonic

Thoracic region: clavicle, ribs and intercostal muscles, Th1-Th5, Th5-Th10; Th10-L2

Lumbosacral dysfunction

Pelvic congestion

Techniques:

Soft tissue techniques and fascial techniques

Muscle energy techniques and positional release techniques HVLA

Long lever techniques

Visceral techniques on the greater and lesser omentum and radix techniques, grand abdominal manoeuvre

Doming diaphragm

Rib raising

Cranial techniques

Findings form for osteopathic treatment Date Case 5

Medical history form was completed by each participant (see Appendix A Medical history form) No immediate contraindications to manual treatment could be identified. Gender: Male Age: 34 years Height: 179 cm Weight: 75 kg

Hypothesis 1: Does a 15-minute osteopathic treatment have an effect on lung function or on the subjective perception of exertion and dyspnoea?

Tick off standardised procedure after completion:

Findings:

Static and dynamic inspection Standing – sitting – supine

Special tests:

Provocation tests (complaint structure):

Palpation:

Oscillation test (somatic dysfunction of the spine, identification of segments):

Breathing movement test (number of breathing cycles, thoracic movement, diaphragm)

Intervention in the subsystems:

Craniosacral system

P.A.M

Rhythm Force Symmetry Amplitude

Visceral system

Subdiaphragmatic central lateral/left lateral right/right

Small pelvis

Parietal system

Cervical region: occiput, upper cervical spine, respiratory accessory muscles hypertonic

Thoracic region: clavicle, ribs and intercostal muscles, Th1-Th5, Th5-Th10; Th10-L2

Lumbosacral dysfunction

Pelvic congestion

Techniques:

Soft tissue techniques and fascial techniques

Muscle energy techniques and positional release techniques HVLA

Long lever techniques

Visceral techniques on the greater and lesser omentum and radix techniques, grand abdominal manoeuvre

Doming diaphragm

Rib raising

Cranial techniques

Findings sheet for osteopathic treatment Date Case 6

Medical history form was completed by each participant (see Appendix A Medical history form) No immediate contraindications to manual treatment could be identified. Gender: Male Age: 26 years Height: 182 cm Weight: 82 kg

Hypothesis 1: Does a 15-minute osteopathic treatment have an effect on lung function or on the subjective perception of exertion and dyspnoea?

Check off standardised procedure after completion:

Findings:

Static and dynamic inspection Standing – sitting – supine

Special tests:

Provocation tests (complaint structure):

Palpation:

Oscillation test (somatic dysfunction of the spine, identification of segments):

Breathing movement test (number of breathing cycles, thoracic movement, diaphragm)

Intervention in the subsystems:

Craniosacral system

P.A.M

Rhythm Force Symmetry Amplitude

Visceral system

Subdiaphragmatic central lateral/left lateral right/right

Small pelvis

Parietal system

Cervical region: occiput, upper cervical spine, respiratory accessory muscles hypertonic

Thoracic region: clavicle, ribs and intercostal muscles, Th1-Th5, Th5-Th10; Th10-L2

Lumbosacral dysfunction

Pelvic congestion

Techniques:

Soft tissue techniques and fascial techniques

Muscle energy techniques and positional release techniques HVLA

Long lever techniques

Visceral techniques on the greater and lesser omentum and radix techniques, grand abdominal manoeuvres

Doming diaphragm

Rib raising

Cranial techniques

Findings form for osteopathic treatment Date Case 7

Medical history form was completed by each participant (see Appendix A Medical history form) No immediate contraindications to manual treatment could be identified. Gender: Male Age: 22 years Height: 75 cm Weight: 75 kg

Hypothesis 1: Does a 15-minute osteopathic treatment have an effect on lung function or on the subjective perception of exertion and dyspnoea?

Check off standardised procedure after completion:

Findings:

Static and dynamic inspection Standing – sitting – supine

Special tests:

Provocation tests (complaint structure):

Palpation:

Oscillation test (somatic dysfunction of the spine, identification of segments):

Breathing movement test (number of breathing cycles, thoracic movement, diaphragm)

Intervention in the subsystems:

Craniosacral system

P.A.M

Rhythm Force Symmetry Amplitude

Visceral system

Subdiaphragmatic central lateral/left lateral right/right

Small pelvis

Parietal system

Cervical region: occiput, upper cervical spine, respiratory accessory muscles hypertonic

Thoracic region: clavicle, ribs and intercostal muscles, Th1-Th5, Th5-Th10; Th10-L2

Lumbosacral dysfunction

Pelvic congestion

Techniques:

Soft tissue techniques and fascial techniques

Muscle energy techniques and positional release techniques HVLA

Long lever techniques

Visceral techniques on the greater and lesser omentum and radix techniques, grand abdominal manoeuvres

Doming diaphragm

Rib raising

Cranial techniques

Findings sheet for osteopathic treatment Date Case 8

Medical history form was completed by each participant (see Appendix A Medical history form) No immediate contraindications to manual treatment could be identified. Gender: Female Age: 26 years Height: 56 kg Weight: 163 cm

Hypothesis 1: Does a 15-minute osteopathic treatment have an effect on lung function or, using the , on subjective feelings of exertion and dyspnoea?

Check off standardised procedure after completion:

Findings:

Static and dynamic inspection Standing – sitting – supine

Special tests:

Provocation tests (complaint structure):

Palpation:

Oscillation test (somatic dysfunction of the spine, identification of segments):

Breathing movement test (number of breathing cycles, thoracic movement, diaphragm)

Intervention in the subsystems:

Craniosacral system

P.A.M

Rhythm Force Symmetry Amplitude

Visceral system

Subdiaphragmatic central lateral/left lateral right/right

Small pelvis

Parietal system

Cervical region: occiput, upper cervical spine, respiratory accessory muscles hypertonic

Thoracic region: clavicle, ribs and intercostal muscles, Th1-Th5, Th5-Th10; Th10-L2

Lumbosacral dysfunction

Pelvic congestion

Techniques:

Soft tissue techniques and fascial techniques

Muscle energy techniques and positional release techniques HVLA

Long lever techniques

Visceral techniques on the greater and lesser omentum and radix techniques, grand abdominal manoeuvre

Doming diaphragm

Rib raising

Cranial techniques

Findings form for osteopathic treatment Date Case 9

Medical history form was completed by each participant (see Appendix A Medical history form) No immediate contraindications to manual treatment could be identified. Gender: Female Age: 21 years Height: 165 cm Weight: 52 kg

Hypothesis 1: Does a 15-minute osteopathic treatment have an effect on lung function or on the subjective perception of exertion and dyspnoea?

Check off standardised procedure after completion:

Findings:

Static and dynamic inspection Standing – sitting – supine

Special tests:

Provocation tests (complaint structure):

Palpation:

Oscillation test (somatic dysfunction of the spine, identification of segments):

Breathing movement test (number of breathing cycles, thoracic movement, diaphragm)

Intervention in the subsystems:

Craniosacral system

P.A.M

Rhythm Force Symmetry Amplitude

Visceral system

Subdiaphragmatic central lateral/left lateral right/right

Small pelvis

Parietal system

Cervical region: occiput, upper cervical spine, respiratory accessory muscles hypertonic

Thoracic region: clavicle, ribs and intercostal muscles, Th1-Th5, Th5-Th10; Th10-L2

Lumbosacral dysfunction

Pelvic congestion

Techniques:

Soft tissue techniques and facial techniques

Muscle energy techniques and positional release techniques HVLA

Long lever techniques

Visceral techniques on the greater and lesser omentum and radix techniques, grand abdominal manoeuvre

Doming diaphragm

Rib raising

Cranial techniques

Findings sheet for osteopathic treatment Date Case 10

Medical history form was completed by each participant (see Appendix A Medical history form) No immediate contraindications to manual treatment could be identified. Gender: Female Age: 27 years Height: 165 cm Weight: 48 kg

Hypothesis 1: Does a 15-minute osteopathic treatment have an effect on lung function or on the subjective perception of exertion and dyspnoea?

Check off standardised procedure after completion:

Findings:

Static and dynamic inspection Standing – sitting – supine

Special tests:

Provocation tests (complaint structure):

Palpation:

Oscillation test (somatic dysfunction of the spine, identification of segments):

Breathing movement test (number of breathing cycles, thoracic movement, diaphragm)

Intervention in the subsystems:

Craniosacral system

P.A.M

Rhythm Force Symmetry Amplitude

Visceral system

Subdiaphragmatic central lateral/left lateral right/right

Small pelvis

Parietal system

Cervical region: occiput, upper cervical spine, respiratory accessory muscles hypertonic

Thoracic region: clavicle, ribs and intercostal muscles, Th1-Th5, Th5-Th10; Th10-L2

Lumbosacral dysfunction

Pelvic congestion

Techniques:

Soft tissue techniques and facial techniques

Muscle energy techniques and positional release techniques HVLA

Long lever techniques

Visceral techniques on the greater and lesser omentum and radix techniques, grand abdominal manoeuvre

Doming diaphragm

Rib raising

Cranial techniques

Findings form for osteopathic treatment Date Case 11

Medical history form was completed by each participant (see Appendix A Medical history form) No immediate contraindications for manual treatment could be identified. Gender: Female Age: 20 Height: 170 Weight: 63

Hypothesis 1: Does a 15-minute osteopathic treatment have an effect on lung function or on the subjective perception of exertion and dyspnoea?

Check off standardised procedure after completion:

Findings:

Static and dynamic inspection Standing – sitting – supine

Special tests:

Provocation tests (complaint structure):

Palpation:

Oscillation test (somatic dysfunction of the spine, identification of segments):

Breathing movement test (number of breathing cycles, thoracic movement, diaphragm)

Intervention in the subsystems:

Craniosacral system

P.A.M

Rhythm Force Symmetry Amplitude

Visceral system

Subdiaphragmatic central lateral/left lateral right/right

Small pelvis

Parietal system

Cervical region: occiput, upper cervical spine, respiratory accessory muscles hypertonic

Thoracic region: clavicle, ribs and intercostal muscles, Th1-Th5, Th5-Th10; Th10-L2

Lumbosacral dysfunction

Pelvic congestion

Techniques:

Soft tissue techniques and facial techniques

Muscle energy techniques and positional release techniques HVLA

Long lever techniques

Visceral techniques on the greater and lesser omentum and radix techniques, grand abdominal manoeuvre

Doming diaphragm

Rib raising

Cranial techniques

Findings form for osteopathic treatment Date Case 12

Medical history form was completed by each participant (see Appendix A Medical history form) No immediate contraindications to manual treatment could be identified. Gender: Female Age: 20 years Height: 173 cm Weight: 65 kg

Hypothesis 1: Does a 15-minute osteopathic treatment have an effect on lung function or on the subjective perception of exertion and dyspnoea?

Tick off standardised procedure after completion:

Findings:

Static and dynamic inspection Standing – sitting – supine

Special tests:

Provocation tests (complaint structure):

Palpation:

Oscillation test (somatic dysfunction of the spine, identification of segments):

Breathing movement test (number of breathing cycles, thoracic movement, diaphragm)

Intervention in the subsystems:

Craniosacral system

P.A.M

Rhythm Force Symmetry Amplitude

Visceral system

Subdiaphragmatic central lateral/left lateral right/right

Small pelvis

Parietal system

Cervical region: occiput, upper cervical spine, respiratory accessory muscles hypertonic

Thoracic region: clavicle, ribs and intercostal muscles, Th1-Th5, Th5-Th10; Th10-L2

Lumbosacral dysfunction

Pelvic congestion

Techniques:

Soft tissue techniques and fascial techniques

Muscle energy techniques and positional release techniques HVLA

Long lever techniques

Visceral techniques on the greater and lesser omentum and radix techniques, grand abdominal manoeuvres

Doming diaphragm

Rib raising

Cranial techniques

Findings form for osteopathic treatment Date Case 13

Medical history form was completed by each participant (see Appendix A Medical history form) No immediate contraindications to manual treatment could be identified. Gender: Female Age: 21 years Height: 162 cm Weight: 51 kg

Hypothesis 1: Does a 15-minute osteopathic treatment have an effect on lung function or on the subjective perception of exertion and dyspnoea?

Check off standardised procedure after completion:

Findings:

Static and dynamic inspection Standing – sitting – supine

Special tests:

Provocation tests (complaint structure):
Palpation:
Oscillation test (somatic dysfunction of the spine, identification of segments):
Breathing movement test (number of breathing cycles, thoracic movement, diaphragm)
Intervention in the subsystems:
Craniosacral system
P.A.M
Rhythm Force Symmetry Amplitude
Visceral system
Subdiaphragmatic central lateral/left lateral right/right
Small pelvis
Parietal system
Cervical region: occiput, upper cervical spine, respiratory accessory muscles hypertonic
Thoracic region: clavicle, ribs and intercostal muscles, Th1-Th5, Th5-Th10; Th10-L2
Lumbosacral dysfunction
Pelvic congestion
Techniques:
Soft tissue techniques and fascial techniques
Muscle energy techniques and positional release techniques HVLA
Long lever techniques
Visceral techniques on the greater and lesser omentum and radix techniques, grand abdominal manoeuvre
Doming diaphragm
Rib raising
Cranial techniques

Findings form for osteopathic treatment Date Case 14

Medical history form was completed by each participant (see Appendix A Medical history form) No immediate contraindications to manual treatment could be identified. Gender: Female Age: 20 years Height: 183 cm Weight: 85 kg

Hypothesis 1: Does a 15-minute osteopathic treatment have an effect on lung function or on the subjective perception of exertion and dyspnoea?

Check off standardised procedure after completion:
Findings:
Static and dynamic inspection Standing – sitting – supine
Special tests:
Provocation tests (complaint structure):
Palpation:
Oscillation test (somatic dysfunction of the spine, identification of segments):
Breathing movement test (number of breathing cycles, thoracic movement, diaphragm)
Intervention in the subsystems:

Craniosacral system

P.A.M

Rhythm Force Symmetry Amplitude

Visceral system

Subdiaphragmatic central lateral/left lateral right/right

Small pelvis

Parietal system

Cervical region: occiput, upper cervical spine, respiratory accessory muscles hypertonic

Thoracic region: clavicle, ribs and intercostal muscles, Th1-Th5, Th5-Th10; Th10-L2

Lumbosacral dysfunction

Pelvic congestion

Techniques:

Soft tissue techniques and fascial techniques

Muscle energy techniques and positional release techniques HVLA

Long lever techniques

Visceral techniques on the greater and lesser omentum and radix techniques, grand abdominal manoeuvre

Doming diaphragm

Rib raising

Cranial techniques

Control group

Findings sheet for microwave (placebo) treatment, cases 1–10

Only one findings sheet is shown as an example for these 10 participants, as no further findings were recorded.

All participants were observed by a therapist with their upper body naked and lying on their stomach for a period of 15 minutes after the inactive microwave was installed.

The medical history form was completed by each participant (see Appendix A Medical History Form). No immediate contraindications to microwave (placebo) treatment were identified.

Gender: male/female

Age

Height

Weight

Hypothesis 1: What effect does this intervention have on lung function and on subjective feelings of exertion and dyspnoea?

FSC
www.fsc.org
MIX
Papier | Fördert
gute Waldnutzung
FSC® C083411

Kolibri 360 GmbH
Ferdinand-Jühlke-Straße 7
99095 Erfurt, Deutschland
produktsicherheit@kolibri360.de

Druck:
CPI Druckdienstleistungen GmbH
im Auftrag der
Kolibri 360 GmbH
Ferdinand-Jühlke-Str. 7
99095 Erfurt